THE REGENERATION OF ALEXANDRIA'S PURPOSE

I found my life purpose by asking questions, failing, and making a path that only made sense to me. - Alexandria Williams

I was never your average sports star when growing up. I played multiple sports but never fully committed to just one. Whatever I wanted to do or try, I did. I loved the idea of being in various sports or trying out new fitness regimens, as it never got boring. You might say I had commitment issues, but I believed in trying something at least once before disregarding it.

As a teenage girl, the only things I can say I committed to were simply graduating from college preparatory high school—because it cost an insane amount of money—and helping my grandmother, who is a stroke survivor, learn how to adjust to her meals after it was confirmed she was diabetic. This was the focus of my teenage commitment until I hit my twenties.

Because of my early interest in multiple sports, it's no surprise that a decade later I found myself interested in multi-distance sports such as triathlons and duathlons. When I was twenty-five, I competed in my first duathlon. A duathlon involves an athlete running for a period of time, then biking for an extensive number miles, then insanely hopping off the bike only to run again for a period of time to hopefully cross the finish line and receive a banana, apple, medal, or cheering.

On my first duathlon, I unfortunately failed to complete the entire duathlon, as I missed the cutoff time for completion by five minutes. That cause me to be depressed for what seemed like a period of almost a month. I don't like the feeling of failing, and I am very hard on myself, so this was torture for me. Eventually, I got tired of my mind replaying the "oh if only I had *(insert the many other things I could have done)*" and sulking. Therefore, I vowed to go all out and compete in a triathlon.

Now, a triathlon is where an athlete shells out a lot more money than in a duathlon, to swim for a period of time in either a pool, lake, or ocean, then bike for an extensive number of miles, then insanely hop off the bike only to run for some miles to hopefully cross the finish line and receive a banana, apple, medal, foil-like sheet, and cheering. This goal meant that at age twenty-five, I, Alexandria Williams, had to learn how to swim for the first time in my life.

Once I make a goal, you can't stop me. Plus, I lucked out, as my boss, Mary, was an Ironman champion. An Ironman competition is deemed to be the hardest type of triathlon, so hard that it has its own name. Anyhow, she helped me find a local swimming class at the community college. I faithfully took every swimming lesson that was offered, while facing my fear of large pools of water, and I indirectly found calmness within the pool. From this point onward, researching and learning everything pertaining to swimming, biking, and running took up my days and nights.

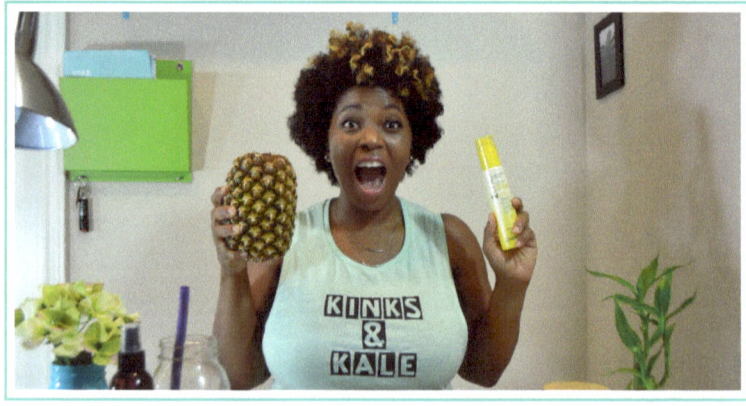

However, on my journey toward being a triathlete, I kept hitting a major but unexpected roadblock. I had to tackle head-on—literally and figuratively speaking—how to deal with what was becoming a huge mess on my head: my former straight, thick hair. Yeah, my hair was holding me back. I was in the pool four times a week for the first time in my life, and I had no idea what to do with my hair. What was a sista who had a head full of thick hair and a full-time corporate job, and who was restricted by a budget, supposed to do? The solution to this problem was simple: go research and figure it out—quickly.

THE EASIEST WAY
TO SOLVE A PROBLEM
IS TO RESEARCH,
LISTEN AND FIGURE IT
OUT - QUICKLY.

———

ALEXANDRIA WILLIAMS

My journey into FitHair started at this moment. The seed was planted as I was learning the mechanics of swimming and the direct impact of proper foods to eat. In addition, I also had to learn how to manage my hair as I pursued this new endeavor. This meant lots of trial and error with different hairstyles and products. I researched a lot and discussed with cosmetologists for advice on product creation and basic knowledge of hair structure so that I could create my own hair products or tweak purchased ones to better suit my specific needs.

Pause. To give you a context of what I was working with back then, you have to understand the beauty industry. Carol's Daughter, now a million-dollar company and a part of the L'Oreal brand, had just entered the Dallas market in three stores; Fashionbomb.com, which is one of the most influential blogs in today's fashion game, had just been launched a year earlier; and Instagram was still in the making and virtually unknown to many of us.

Nowadays, you can simply rush to Target to grab popular natural hair products like Jane Carter, The Mane Choice, Giovanni, and Oyin Handmane hair products. You can also go online to research and compare products or to watch a YouTube video, and within five minutes you have access to the right steps, products, and much more on how you can maintain your hair. The current generation is truly blessed, so understand the frustrations I had back then when I had neither the access nor the knowledge to facilitate the achievement of my goal.

ANYWAY... LETS GET BACK TO THE STORY.

Months later, I was able to compete in my first triathlon and *finish*. It wasn't the best finish, but I did it and fell in love with the sport; however, my hair consistently kept getting in my way. I eventually decided to cut off all my chemically treated hair and let my coils free. (This is known as a "big chop." Google it to get a better understanding.) I am going to be honest, I didn't like my short, coily hair, and therefore I was forced to learn everything I could about wigs. I covered up my short hair immediately after working out with a big curly wig without shame.

As my training intensified, I started getting questions on a daily basis from folks at the gym. Countless men and women approached me as I was swimming, running, or hopping on a bike. There wasn't a day that went by that I wasn't asked about my hair regimen or workout plans. I met so many women who had been in my situation: they had been afraid to swim for fear they would mess up their hair in the pool. Answering their questions or finding solutions that could help them sparked my passion to help them remove the barriers that were standing in their way to being healthy and fit.

As I began to speak and write about these issues, I found a passion in it and started blogging on how I could solve these problems. Then a year or so later, I hit another major roadblock after having completed a number of triathlons. My entire body experienced an allergic reaction to something I knew nothing about, and the doctors had no idea what was causing it. While most people would get scared, the only thing that ran through my mind was, "I still have to work out, since I just paid $150 for a tri that is coming up in a few months."

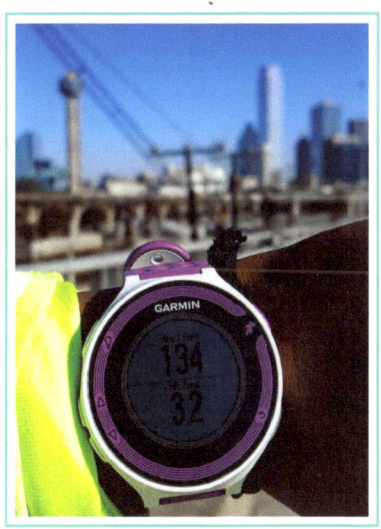

Training helped me maintain my sanity during a time when anything I put in my mouth or on my skin could trigger a reaction that could land me in the hospital. It was exhausting having to write down everything I ate, drank, and used daily. The details of writing down my daily habits were intense. It wasn't just, "I had a #1 from Whataburger," but more like **EVERY INGREDIENT** in **EVERYTHING**, and I mean **EVERYTHING. EVERY SINGLE THING**. A #1 meal from any fast food stop typically filled a page in my journal just from all the ingredients. During this time, I had to Google and research for information from any available resources, as I didn't have a readily-available complete ingredient list.

In the process of looking up ingredients, I was amazed at how something as simple as a bun or flavored drink contained ingredients I had never known of. After evaluating my diet, the doctor suggested that I should switch to a simple diet that contained foods like meat, rice, broccoli, etc., so that it would be possible to find out the foods that might have been responsible for triggering my allergic reaction. I happily agreed because I was tired of writing a long list of complex ingredients for every item I used each day.

For about three months, I keenly observed what I put in my mouth, as well as what I applied on my skin. I took note of any changes to the reaction and my body. Surprisingly, I realized how certain foods had a positive effect on me. After avoiding foods and products that had harmful ingredients, I felt more energetic, and I noticed a positive change in my skin, as well as faster recovery after workouts. I also noticed a change in my mood despite everything that was happening to me.

On top of this, my hair also grew thicker than before. This was very fascinating to me, and it prompted me to read books and consult vitamin managers at Whole Foods, Sprouts and Natural Grocers so as to learn about supplements and the breakdown process of certain foods.

Eventually, while in my new periodontitis office, I answered a million other health-related questions that were basically written out in a notebook. The doctor couldn't confirm the problem, nor did the tests he conducted. Therefore, he began to inquire about my simple daily habits. These habits include sleeping, washing my face, brushing my teeth, etc. We went into the details of brushing my teeth, such as when I did it, what type of mouthwash I used, how long I used it, how many times a day I brushed my teeth during that week, and much more. Pretty detailed, right?

After much pondering, he noticed something new I had introduced into my brushing routine: my brand of toothpaste. Because the price of my normal toothpaste had increased to seven dollars, I switched to a cheaper brand I had used in college. As simple as it seemed, it was the culprit to my allergic reaction. **"ARE YOU KIDDING ME!"** was the thought that crossed my mind. I immediately stopped using this cheap brand and went back to good ole faithful, and the reaction went away. I also googled the cheap toothpaste and saw countless comments from folks discussing how they had experienced the same problem.

My heart sank, and like them, I got pissed beyond a doubt as to how this could be legal. I hated that my frugalness had led to hundreds of dollars in doctors' bills, hours of wasted time, and self-esteem issues from the embarrassment of having puffy lips, Starbucks-red-cup gums, and some weight gain from the prescribed steroids. However, in the midst of my frustration, I saw the positive. I had benefited so much from acquiring a wealth of knowledge: I learned the direct impact of what I ate, worked out, learned to live holistically, and embraced simplicity. In addition, I completed another triathlon during this time, which made me feel like an official rock star in my mind.

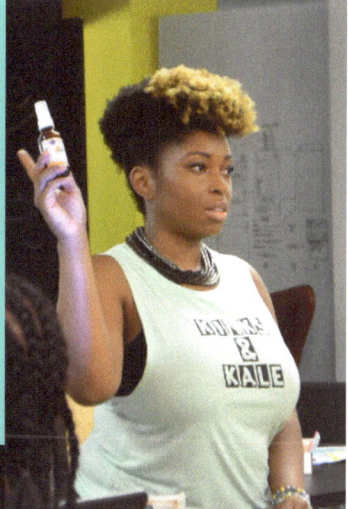

WITH THIS NEW KNOWLEDGE AND EXPERIENCE I VOWED TO MAKE IT MY MISSION TO USE MY WRITING AND VOICE TO EDUCATE PEOPLE ON HOW TO LIVE A HEALTHY LIFE FROM THE INSIDE OUT. THIS BOOK IS A REFLECTION OF MY PASSION AND MISSION.

The **FitHair™ Foundations** isn't your typical book. The book is written not only to serve as a basic guideline for maintaining healthy hair, but also to lay some foundational principles that many people are struggling to find out from reliable and authentic resources. This book doesn't contain a lot of scientific information, nor is its purpose to sell you a bunch of supplements. There are a million books dedicated to "helping you lose weight instantly" or that promise you can take charge of your life by "eating air and omitting a certain food group," which you may have already read. I don't want to waste your money or time on a boring "sales" book.

This book does not fit in that category because that's not my purpose or lane. If you have ever heard me speak at a lecture, workshop, or on a panel, I am very honest with my attendees on health and anything that relates to the beauty industry, but most of all, I have a gift for taking complex information and breaking it down into simple, digestible information. This book is a reflection of that.

To be frank, I have read lots of misleading books, tried many diets, and heard complaints from hundreds of people, so I know there needs to be something different. Something real. Something honest and true that you can read and apply immediately to start getting the results you are struggling with.

SO WITH THAT, LET'S START FROM THE INSIDE AND GET TO IT.

IMAGINE YOURSELF AS A LIVING HOUSE. GOD COMES IN TO REBUILD THAT HOUSE. AT FIRST, PERHAPS, YOU CAN UNDERSTAND WHAT HE IS DOING. HE IS GETTING THE DRAINS RIGHT AND STOPPING THE LEAKS IN THE ROOF AND SO ON; YOU KNEW THAT THOSE JOBS NEEDED DOING AND SO YOU ARE NOT SURPRISED. BUT PRESENTLY HE STARTS KNOCKING THE HOUSE ABOUT IN A WAY THAT HURTS ABOMINABLY AND DOES NOT SEEM TO MAKE ANY SENSE. WHAT ON EARTH IS HE UP TO? THE EXPLANATION IS THAT HE IS BUILDING QUITE A DIFFERENT HOUSE FROM THE ONE YOU THOUGHT OF - THROWING OUT A NEW WING HERE, PUTTING ON AN EXTRA FLOOR THERE, RUNNING UP TOWERS, MAKING COURTYARDS. YOU THOUGHT YOU WERE BEING MADE INTO A DECENT LITTLE COTTAGE: BUT HE IS BUILDING A PALACE. HE INTENDS TO COME AND LIVE IN IT HIMSELF.

———

C.S. Lewis, Mere Christianity

Groundwork

LESSON 01

I really hate discussing my list of accomplishments, and I like to let my work speak for itself. While I have been featured by many different media outlets such as *ABC Nightly News, Dallas Morning News,* and *JET Magazine*; have been elected 2016 Women's Health Action hero; and am nationally known as the **FitHair™expert**, I want to push the accomplishments aside and just be truthful.

I, Alexandria Williams, am not some skinny girl who does yoga, drink nothing but juice everyday, post pretty pictures on the gram (Instagram) of my toned abs and buys burlap purses at Whole Foods. I have seen this carbon copy person within fitness and frankly I thought all fitness and wellness folks were "this type of person." I tried to be "that" type of person and honestly it was a HAWT-MESS. I nearly passed out from dieting and went into my umptenth mid-life crisis. I have friends who drink juice all day, have awesome abs and are Yogis. I love them dearly but this is who they are authentically and they inspire me. However, I cannot and will not be a replica of others.

After trying for years, I got fed up and swore to embrace my flaws, strengths, and all. I had to find out who I was, who I was becoming, who I wasn't, and who I would never be. I had to be okay with it all. I got comfortable with my failures and fears, my internal insecurities, my thick thighs, wide feet, uneven skin tone, and wild hair. The things I hated were ironically the things that made me who I was. Besides, they connected me with so many people who were struggling with the same issues each day. I declared a long time ago to not become a disservice to others by being a replica of something just because it's what folks thought was accepted by society.

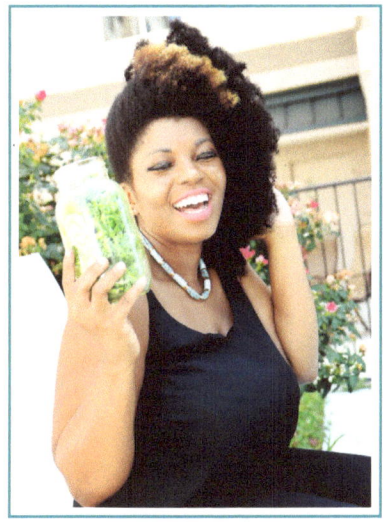

I have experienced a lot in my short years, and my failures have made me look deeper within myself and truly understand who I am and who I am not. While I LOVE kale and green juices, I can also be seen enjoying a gluten-filled white-sugar-cream-filled happiness that is perfectly packaged in a cupcake, while wearing a cheap Marvel T-shirt I purchased at Target, on any given day. It's just who I am, and I am happy with it. The realization of my love of both sugary cupcakes and kale juice led to me focus more on the importance of balance, moderation, and mostly having a solid foundation within one's journey in life.

I have spoken in countless seminars, workshops, and events, and one thing I have learned is that most of the attendees lack proper education on the foundation of not just eating healthy but also the direct impact doing so has on your skin, body, and hair. My goal is to lay a basic foundation of healthy hair from the inside out. Setting a realistic foundation will help change a few small areas you probably need to work on. Once you have started making a few changes, with time you will realize that the journey of health and wellness has a snowball effect. But without the basic and proper foundation, many people end up wasting countless amounts of time and money on trying to find a product that solves something it can't solve. Especially in the beauty industry, the importance of having a proper foundation should not be underestimated. One has to be realistic with their goals. I won't preach too much or go into great detail because let's face it, you're probably stressing right now on what to eat, or otherwise wondering whether you will have enough time to read this book.

And don't worry, I am not judging you at all if you're reading this while eating a Big Mac, with some super-size fries and a Diet Coke on the side. The only thing I will judge you for is that you probably aren't having this with the greatness of a Whataburger and Dr. Pepper, which are true Texan Life Essentials. (I am a Texan girl. What can I say?) All jokes aside, keep in mind that this is a judge-free zone as you continue reading.

Before moving on further, let's agree on one thing: At the end of the day, make sure you are doing what's best for you. Please consult your doctors, dietitians, folks in the scrubs, chiropractor, church members, or whoever is your primary health advisor, because you know yourself better than I do. I am not trying to have anyone putting blame on me because they strictly followed my advice and passed out because they failed to take their prescribed daily meds.

I am writing this as I am unemployed and transitioning to working for myself fully. This means I have pennies, a small 401k, and some prayers. The thought of someone attempting to sue me because "in your book you told me to drink a smoothie and I got sick" will put me in a state of a sleeping beauty coma until the day Jesus saves me from the Rapture. Take this as your disclaimer, or check out the legal one at the end of the book.

TAKEAWAY:

GROUNDWORK IS A TIME TO ESTABLISH BASIC PRINCIPLES OR A GOOD FOUNDATION BEFORE YOU EMBARK ON A NEW GOAL OR JOURNEY.

TODAY I AM A GREEN SMOOTHIE, 1/2 DONUT,
AMY'S LASAGNA FROZEN DINNER, 35 PISTACHIO,
1/2 GLAZED DONUT, CHICK-FIL-A FRENCH FRIES,
SIDE SALAD AND A SWEET TEA.

———

Alexandria Williams

You Are What You Eat
LESSON 02

Growing up, I didn't have the luxury of enjoying cable TV. Any cable TV channels that I watched were when I visited my cousins and my Aunt Helen and Uncle Gary. They had ALL the channels back then, and frankly, they still do to this day. Thus, my cousins, who are like siblings to me, all grew up thinking cable was standard on all TVs.

I, on the other hand, grew up in the hood—Oak Cliff, which was a small area outside of downtown Dallas. My childhood was like a younger black version of *The Golden Girls*, but set in the "urban" area of Dallas. My grandmother, mom, and I all lived in a two-bedroom house until my mom and I moved out as I entered high school. I attended a very expensive college preparatory school through a scholarship (no not an athletic scholarship—three snaps in a circle) where books were easily $1,500 a semester and the kids drove better cars than most teachers.

The thought of asking for cable never crossed my mind, because that "cable money" was spent on private school tuition (it wasn't a full ride), approved school shoes, and the goodness of Hy-Top packaged goods. We didn't have many channels, but the one I enjoyed the most was PBS.

PBS was my favorite because the channel was always crystal clear and had my favorite shows, such as *Ghostwriter* and *Magic School Bus*. One afternoon, I watched an episode of *Magic School Bus* that altered my foundation of how I looked at food.

On this particular episode, one of the students, named Arnold, was complaining because his skin was orange in color. Miss Frizzle, the class teacher, together with the class, gathered to magically go inside Arnold's body to figure out why he was turning orange. Eventually, the students learned Arnold's skin was turning orange because he had been eating seaweed wraps nonstop for a few weeks. It was odd because seaweed is dark green, but he was turning orange.

After researching and exploring his body for some time, the class learned the seaweed wraps were actually carrots (orange) wrapped in a thin sheet of seaweed paper (dark green.) Arnold was turning orange because he kept eating mostly carrots. Carrots are filled with beta-carotene and are the color orange. Even without scientific background, you learn that Arnold's habit of eating nothing but carrots made his skin turn orange (or as I thought the first time I watched it, he was becoming a carrot).

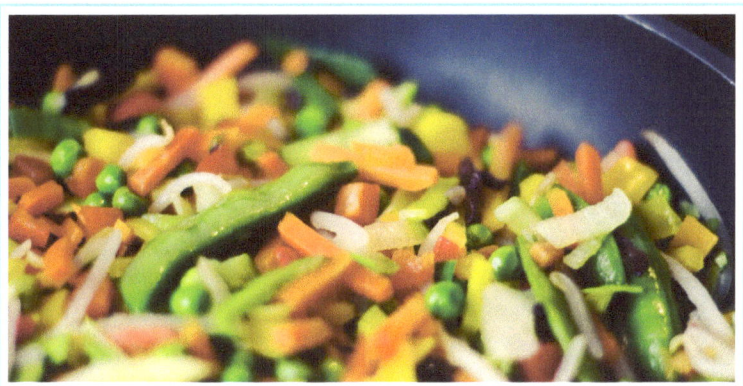

And just like that, along with millions of other kids, I learned the basic principle, "You are what you eat." Just like Arnold, whatever you are consuming will become a part of you. While I don't mind the thought of turning into a cupcake, I know the true error of this thought, and the damage of eating one too many cupcakes. Cupcakes are awesome, but we can't live on just cupcakes alone, unless they are salad cupcakes, juice cupcakes, broccoli cupcakes, etc. You get the picture.

Eh . . . grownup example.

So if you didn't understand the Magic School Bus reference or simply don't believe Miss Frizzle's awesomeness, I will use an adult "real-life" example. For employment, many businesses require a background check and a drug test. With my last employer in corporate America, I had to complete a drug test before I was allowed to start working. When I arrived to take my drug test, the technician asked me what type of drug test I wanted to take. I was confused by the question of what type. I thought you just peed in a cup and went on about your life. The technician explained to me that there were a variety of ways they tested for drugs, such as urine, blood, hair, saliva, and sweat.

I had no idea there were so many ways to test for drugs, but the one that stood out was the one with hair. The tech informed me, "Many people who are recovering or currently on drugs tend to shave their heads in order to avoid the hair follicle test because the hair can show a blueprint of what's going on internally, which includes usage of drugs." I never thought I would learn so much by simply going to pee in a cup. The idea of folks being bald to avoid detection of drugs really surprised me. I wondered if that one time I had second-hand weed smoke at a college party would show up in my hair follicle drug test. Luckily, I wasn't required to provide a sample of my hair; I just had to provide a urine sample.

It is with this new knowledge that I wondered what else a strand of hair could show, outside of the drugs. I eventually searched online, and soon learned that hair could highlight a variety of internal and external factors in a person. Your body needs a variety of nutrients, vitamins, and minerals in order to function properly. The main way it achieves this is by consuming food. (Yes, rest, hydration, and air are also vital, but I am focusing on food for now.) If you don't feed the body what it requires or you feed it unnatural versions of these requirements, this could result in long-term problems such as brittle hair and nails, thinning hair edges, lack of sleep or concentration, weight gain, and much more. So watch what you eat daily. You are what you eat, drink, and breathe, and so is your hair.

TAKEAWAY:

HEALTHY HAIR IS FED FROM THE INSIDE OUT.

ALWAYS DO YOUR BEST. WHAT YOU PLANT
NOW, YOU WILL HARVEST LATER.

———

Og Mandino

Harvesting Healthy Hair
LESSON 03

When a woman is *pregnant*, one of the first things the doctor discusses with the woman is the importance of healthy eating and a balanced diet. Whatever the mother eats, drinks, or lacks usually affects the baby. This is why we women see so many signs in women's washrooms about avoiding drinking while pregnant, and men don't. The same principle applies to plants and animals. Whatever the animal ate and its state, or where the fruit/vegetable is planted, is passed along to us when we consume it. Once we eat food, our body's primary focus is to store, discard, or utilize it.

So what does this mean for your hair? It's fairly simple. The condition of the food you're eating will affect what's passed along not only to your hair but also to your entire body. It is with this understanding that I focus a lot on eating more "alive" fruits, vegetables, and foods than dead foods (animal meats).

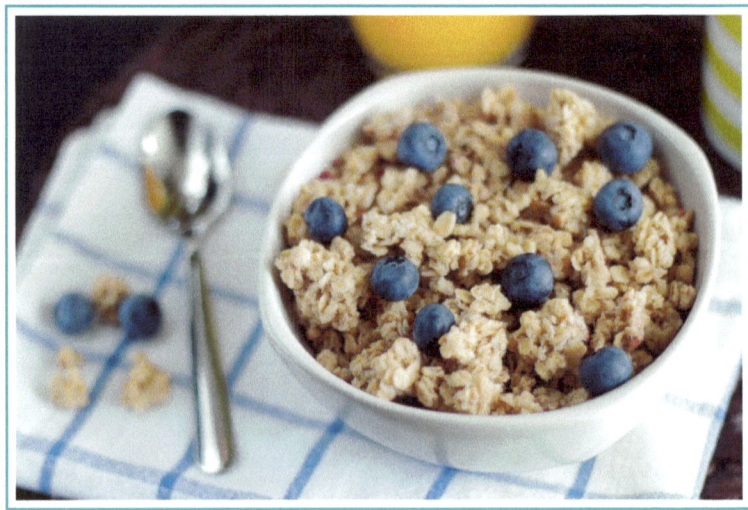

Note: I am not a pro-vegan/pro-vegetarian, nor am I a pro-paleo or whatever the latest diet craze is. What I am pro is eating greens, specifically kale, but I am getting ahead of myself. This book doesn't bash any lifestyle except one that's full of stress and bad vibes and lacking balance.

Back to talking about hair, the actual hair strands we see and feel each day are technically dead. Once they are pushed out of the scalp, they are considered dead. Thus, in order to affect or alter or address the hair, you must take action before the hair is pushed out of your scalp. Before hair is pushed out of the scalp, it's alive and is in the process of gathering vitamins and minerals from our blood cells. Laying a healthy foundation or rich soil will help your body to pass along healthy nutrients to your hair, just like a mother does to her child. You are literally the "mother" of your hair follicles, so feed those babies healthy foods.

TAKEAWAY:

DEVELOPING HEALTHY EATING HABITS WILL RESULT IN HEALTHY HAIR.

FOCUS ON THE END INSTEAD OF THE BEGINNING
AND YOU CAN MAKE STEPS TOWARDS ACHIEVING
WHAT YOU WANT IN THE END.

———

Anthony "Tony" Reed

The Starting Point is the Finishing Line

LESSON 04

As a runner—well, marathoner—and board member of the National Black Marathon Association, I get the pleasure and honor of learning a lot from some amazing, unknown influential athletes in the running community. I have met so many amazing people, from Olympian and Boston Marathon winner Meb Keflezighi, to the first black female marathoner, Marilyn Bevins.

However, Anthony "Tony" Reed is one of the most influential runners who has impacted my life thus far. He is one of the most down-to-earth people I know, yet his resume and list of accomplishments are probably longer than three copies of this book. To the public, he is a history maker and the first African American to run a marathon on all seven continents. But to me, he is the person who connected me to the world of marathons and also registered me for my first and most gruesome marathon. He made the exhaustion of finishing my first marathon disappear by graciously putting around my neck my first marathon finisher's medal, in the middle of pouring rain. He is someone I have dubbed to be my Running Godfather, so to speak.

While Tony has taught me a lot about running and tons of life lessons, one tip that is guarded in my heart and mind is one of our discussions on how to properly train for a marathon. He taught me to think about the end instead of the beginning:

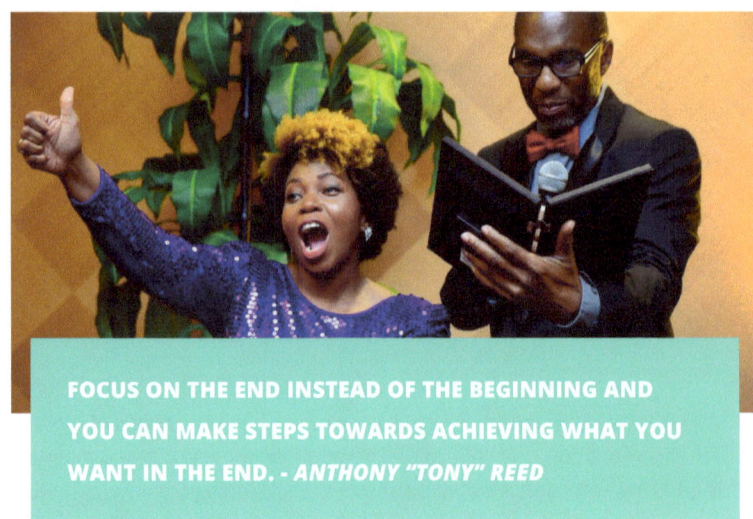

FOCUS ON THE END INSTEAD OF THE BEGINNING AND YOU CAN MAKE STEPS TOWARDS ACHIEVING WHAT YOU WANT IN THE END. - *ANTHONY "TONY" REED*

The true starting point is the goal or the end of a race. Each step you make to achieve your goal is like a check box on your to-do list. Having the finish line in mind helps you create a plan that will support your ultimate goal. No experienced runner just says they don't know what they are running each day. Most runners start with their race dates in mind and create a schedule that is in line with the goal. The vision of the end is the beginning of the journey.

If your ultimate goal is to have healthy hair, you have to accept you will have to make some changes in order to have the results you seek. You have to see the finish line as obtaining healthy hair but embrace various steps and training that need to take place prior to you reaching the intended goal. You have to establish a good foundation and consume healthier foods than the ones you are probably used to. In addition, plan on being consistent in order to achieve your goal of healthier hair. This book is to serve as your foundation and guide to achieving that goal.

TAKEAWAY:

THE JOURNEY TO HEALTHY HAIR STARTS NOW

FOR EVERYTHING THERE IS A SEASON.

———

Ecclesiastes 3:1

ONE DAY I HOPE THE HEALTHCARE SYSTEM
WOULD ALLOW MY DOCTOR TO PRESCRIBE A SPA
DAY OR VACATION.

———

Alexandria Williams

A Balanced Life
LESSON 05

I understand how "normal" it is to work in multiple jobs, go on failed date number 176, take care of your family, cook, clean, and attend networking functions, only to end up sitting in a corner complaining while you empty the bottles of free booze and ultimately get to make the most out of the really-good lighting to post a picture of you looking cute on Instagram. I get it. I am here to tell you for your hair's sake, that running 110 mph every single day does more harm than good. Why? Because the energy and vitamins your body needs to sustain healthy hair, often can be redirected to replace depleted minerals from running at 110 mph every single day.

Extreme stress negatively impacts your hair. Many people who go through stressful events—whether good or bad—such as a loss of a job, divorce, or even the birth of a baby, often experience changes in their hair such as hair loss, thinning edges, shedding, and much more. Again, I am not trying to be your nutritionist and outline everything you should eat, nor am I your therapist to address your stressful events. In all honestly, all I would tell you is that you should take a vacation to the islands and find a place where you can sit down and enjoy God's creation. However, what I will say is this: **balance is critical to your overall wellbeing, and a good balance will help you mentally, spiritually, emotionally, and physically.**

There is nothing wrong with watching a documentary, eating, sleeping, drinking water, or running. All these things are considered by most folks to be good for the human body and soul. However, if you overdo any of these activities, such as binge-watching TV, drinking too much water, or running every day, you will experience TONS of problems. Create sufficient time to rest when training, or simply enjoy a little bit of chocolate every now and then. You don't have to overdo everything. Modify the stressful and become "restful." Find balance in your life.

Establishing balance and eating healthy doesn't mean eating a "balanced" diet of fast foods from a chain of food stores each week by not eating at the same ones every day. It starts by having the proper amounts of nutrition and meals to nourish your hair and body on a daily basis. Make it a habit to review the foods you're consuming each week. Instead of having an entire chocolate bar, try having only a snack-size amount each day. Try swapping out your fried chicken strips with making your own grilled chicken strips and dipping them into your favorite sauce. Choose to be balanced in your eating as well as in your life.

Even Mother Nature encourages us to eat in balance. This is why we often have a surplus of certain fruits and vegetables each season. How do I know this? Well, outside of my best friend Google, if you study what is on sale at the grocery stores during each season, you will come to the same conclusion. Whatever is on sale or super cheap is typically in season.

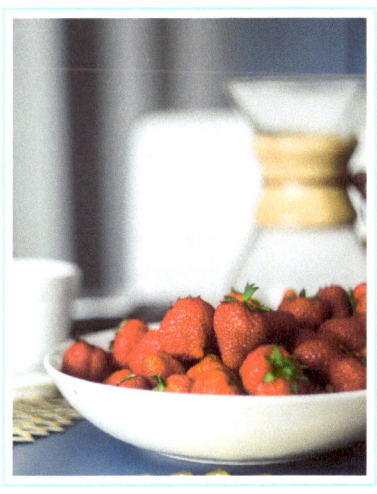

Here is a good example. I love strawberries and grapes. They are about $0.99 a carton in the summer but when winter comes in to Texas, trust me, their price shoots up to $6.99 for the same carton, and the quantity available is much smaller. These fruits are plentiful in the summer, which means they are in their peak season, and they are rare in the wintertime. Grocery stores that have them, often have to ship these items from various parts of the world where they are in season. So instead of overspending during the winter, I opt to switch to frozen fruits or fall back in love with oranges, grapefruits, and red bananas, which are plentiful during the winter.

As you start to establish basic foundations, here are my top five essential habits to having healthy hair and being balanced from the inside out.

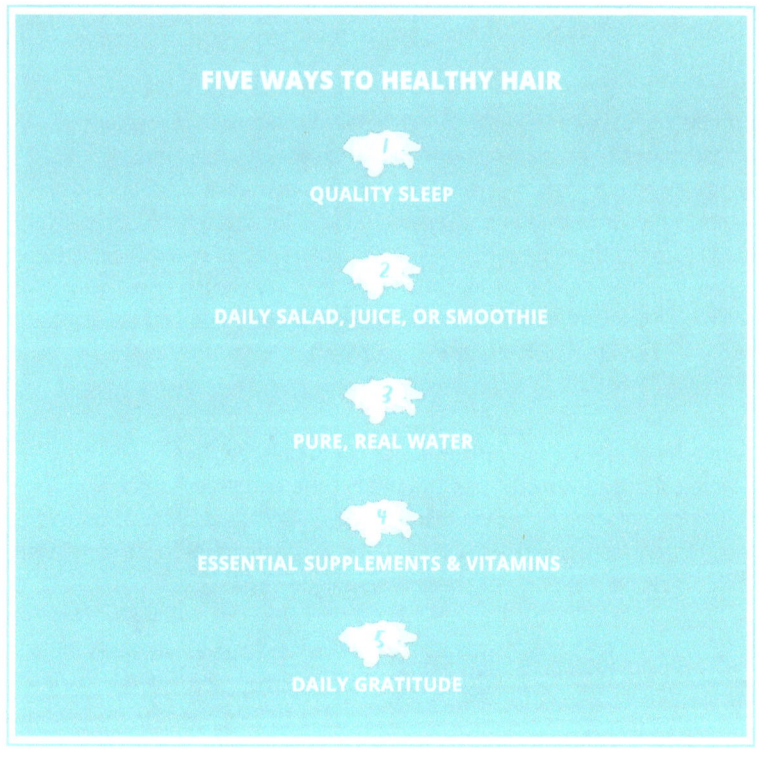

That's it.

If there is anything you can take away from this lesson, it is a principle I live and stand for not just on hair issues but also in life:

TAKEAWAY:

EVERYTHING IN MODERATION, INCLUDING MODERATION. THE SECOND PART IS KEY. DON'T OVER DO IT.

THANKS TO FRUITS AND VEGETABLES, I HAVE
MORE ENERGY, THICKER HAIR, AND MY POOP
DOESN'T SMELL LIKE DEATH.

———

Alexandria Williams

The Root of Health Starts with Digestion
LESSON 06

Have you ever gone into a public restroom and experienced a moment where you ran into a stench which you thought could only be someone about push *Death's* baby out into the toilet? I believe this is a disservice to everyone who walks into the restroom for at least the next half hour. It doesn't seem right to me. I often wonder, if the spirit of Christ is to live within us and we are his temples, what gas mask does the Holy Ghost use to survive the daily decaying of funk that folks push out?

In the previous lesson, I explained that the end is the beginning. This principle applies on the road to healthy hair. If you are what you eat, you have to take the time to figure out what your body is lacking. Your digestive health is one of the key indicators of your overall health. It is believed that the root of health starts with digestion. Many nutrition companies, doctors, and even health activists often quote "the root of all health lies in the digestive system." I have heard this, but didn't fully understand it until I got a chance to visit and spend time at the Garden of Life Headquarters.

Garden of Life is basically a company made up of food fanatics. On any given day, they can provide a detailed list of the ingredients in any product, where it came from, the soil that the seed was harvested from, and much more for every single product. Very few companies can do what they do, and they should be commended. Now, this isn't a commercial, but I wanted to make a statement about the company; most of the company's products contain some form of probiotics or focus on improving gut health. I was fascinated as to why a company would put so much focus on gut health and the digestive system. I learned this key principle from the Garden of Life folks:

> **ANYTHING YOUR BODY TAKES IN, IT WANTS TO DIGEST IT. THE BODY EITHER USES, STORES, OR DISCARDS, THUS DIGESTION IS CRITICAL AND ESSENTIAL TO OPTIMUM HEALTH AND WELL-BEING.**

This is a simple yet profound principle that sums up the complexity of the body. Digestion health is so critical that most Garden of Life products relate in some way to gut health. The first time I learned about gut health, the first things that came to mind were probiotics and enzymes. Earlier in my life, I used to get sick whenever I ate meats. It just seemed like they didn't agree with my body or I felt sick afterward. One January, I went vegan during a forty-day church fasting period. I noticed on the twentieth day that I had lots of energy and that my digestive system was going for the gold medal.

This was great, but my old habits snuck back in, and I went back to eating meats and unhealthy foods. One day after a massive steak dinner, I felt like I was decaying inside, and could smell it from the inside. While no one else could smell this, the bathroom told a different story. I also noticed that my digestion process had slowed down drastically. I did a bit of research and learned that I wasn't eating enough leafy greens and foods rich in fiber. At this point I learned the importance of probiotics and enzymes within the body.

In the show *How Does It Work?*, the site describes this process as "at any given moment, all of the work being done inside any cell is being done by enzymes."[1] The purpose of an enzyme in a cell is to allow the cell to carry out chemical reactions very quickly. These reactions allow the cell to form new things or to take things apart as needed. This is how a cell grows and reproduces.

I know I lost you there. We are getting technical, but stay with me. The most important thing you should know is that enzymes play a vital role in the entire body, particularly the digestion process. Digestive enzymes break down foods so that our bodies can benefit from the nutrients contained in these foods. If we don't have enough or a wide enough variety of enzymes, it becomes difficult for our bodies to properly function and effectively absorb nutrients we take in.

Dr. Edward Howell, MD, author of the seminal book Enzyme Nutrition[2], was among the first pioneers who began studying the role of enzymes and believed it was important to eat certain raw and fermented foods that are high in enzyme content.

So the steak dinner with fried sides of potatoes, okra, and breads that I had often, simply took a long time to digest because I didn't have sufficient enzymes to help with digestion.

Now what does discussing digestion have to do with hair? I get it. Talking about poop makes no sense, but remember, the end is the beginning. If your body isn't able to digest effectively, then it can't have optimum access to the vitamins, minerals, and nutrients it needs. This will negatively affect your hair.

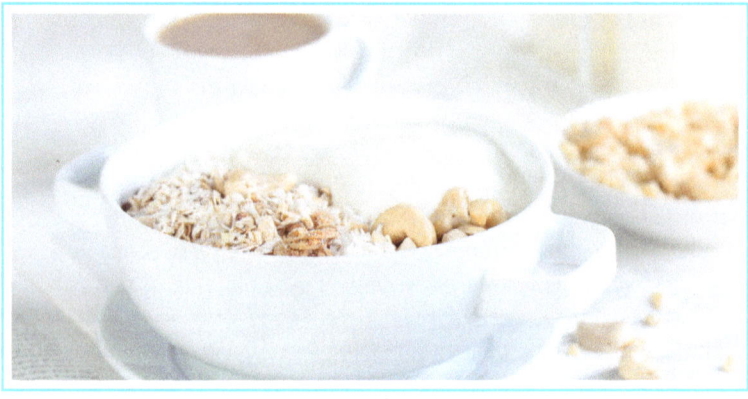

Probiotics are often ignored when it comes to the topic of hair growth. I honestly didn't think they were a vital part of my regimen until I experienced a variety of digestive changes and issues over the last few years. The first step is to make sure you have proper digestive enzymes, which can be found in some of the following foods:

- Cultured vegetables (sauerkraut and kimchi)
- Kefir
- Raw cheese (This is different than traditional cheese.)
- Greek yogurt
- Kombucha

I understand a lot of folks don't like most of these foods or don't have the time to go to stores and get them on a regular basis. So taking a reputable probiotic will work just as well. There are a number of probiotics I would recommend, but if you had to guess, Garden of Life is my number one pick. Nevertheless, having a properly tuned gastrointestinal (gut) tract is key to good health and hair.

TAKEAWAY:

GOOD POOP, ODDLY ENOUGH, CAN LEAD TO GOOD HAIR.

1% OF THE AMERICAN DIET TODAY COMES FROM PROCESSED FOODS (PREDOMINANTLY OILS, SUGAR & FLOUR).

———

Dr. Joel Fuhrmam

Get Ya Juice On
LESSON 07

For some of you, this title might be misleading. Juice today isn't like the juice from a few decades ago. Most juices are filled with preservatives and sugar, which are not only bad for your hair but also for your entire body. The juices most people drink are a package on a shelf and filled with sugar or have a label that says, "Contains 10% real juice." This isn't the juice I am referring to. Juice is a liquid obtained from actual fruits and/or vegetables. For most people, to create healthy juice, you have to have a juicer.

Let's be honest, most people barely have vegetables on a single day. A slice of tomato and lettuce in a BLT, or overcooked green beans in the frozen entrees, is the *normal* amount. Additionally, most people hate vegetables unless they are fried and smothered in oils and fats. Your body needs vegetables, but not the fried kind, and a quick way to incorporate them is by juicing them.

I recommend juicing because juicing allows for more consumption of vitamins and minerals in one serving compared to eating vegetables raw or blending them in a smoothie. You can eat a few handfuls of grapes, but if you were to juice them, you could extract a lot more nutrients than from a few handfuls. Since juicing extracts the fiber, you're able to drink double or triple the amount you might have eaten.

Juicing has been documented and is known to help get rid of sickness, diseases, and much more. To learn more about the benefits of juicing, I highly recommend the movie *Fat, Sick & Nearly Dead*[3] , which chronicles Joe Cross, a morbidly obese man who was stricken with an autoimmune disease. In the documentary, we see Joe attempting to reclaim his health by going on a juice fast for sixty days.

There are countless juicing books, juice fast programs, and juicers currently available in the market; therefore, having a juice a day isn't unattainable. One of my favorite places to grab a juice or smoothie is at a local juice store. I love trying various blends and mixes. When traveling, Jamba Juice is one of my favorite places because they are everywhere in the country. They often let me customize my own juice to meet my nutritional needs while jet setting. From juice sections in the grocery store to making your own at home, there are countless options that allow access to a daily juice. You just have to keep your eyes open.

Vegetables such as kale, swiss chard, celery, and much more are all essential for hair growth, but most people don't like eating them, so juicing is a great option. You can mask the taste of these vegetables with the sweeter fruits you like. If juicing isn't an option, then a packaged green supplement is a quick and portable way of getting your greens. These supplements often contain many different types of greens packaged in powdered or compressed form.
In most cases, green supplements are cheaper than juicing daily and are easier to carry when traveling.

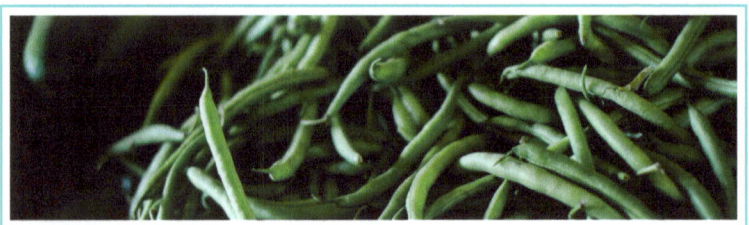

In the end, it doesn't matter if you're steaming a pot of green beans or making a green juice with spinach and mixed fruit, find ways to incorporate vegetables into your daily life. Your hair and body will thank you. To get a few of my favorite picks, you can review my FitHair picks for my favorite green supplements, found in the back of this book.

WE CAN MAKE A COMMITMENT TO PROMOTE VEGETABLES AND FRUITS AND WHOLE GRAINS ON EVERY PART OF EVERY MENU. WE CAN MAKE PORTION SIZES SMALLER AND EMPHASIZE QUALITY OVER QUANTITY. AND WE CAN HELP CREATE A CULTURE - IMAGINE THIS - WHERE OUR KIDS ASK FOR HEALTHY OPTIONS INSTEAD OF RESISTING THEM.

———

Michelle Obama

A Salad a Day Keeps the Doctor Away

LESSON 08

A simple way to stay healthy is to eat salad every day. Salads are filled with tons of fiber and can help keep you lean, trim, and full. The best part about salads is that they are easily available everywhere. From Chick-fil-A to a simple bagged salad at your local grocery store, you can make sure you are staying healthy and are on track anytime of the day. If salads aren't your thing, then have an ice-cold smoothie at the start of your day.

Smoothies are not only easy and affordable but are also a great way to include vitamins, minerals, and vegetables.

I HAVE INCLUDED A FEW SMOOTHIE RECIPES IN THIS BOOK, BUT I WILL PUBLISH A LOT MORE ONLINE. THIS BOOK ISN'T SET TO BE A RECIPE OR FOOD GUIDELINE, SO MAKE SURE YOU KEEP UP WITH ME ONLINE FOR MORE DETAILS AT ALEXANDRIAWILL.COM.

When having salads, try to incorporate more vegetables and less dressing. If you are unsure, try a local restaurant or grocery store salad bar, and try various vegetables, dressings, and fruits. This is an easy way to try out new food combinations.

Avoid high fat and weird dressings that are filled with processed ingredients. If you don't like what is offered, avoid spending money, and figure out for yourself, through trial and error, what works for you. I find having a little bit of vinegar and olive oil and mixing in some seasonings works perfectly on most salads.

If you get in the habit of having a salad every day, you will begin to crave not only salads but also vegetables daily. Make it a habit and try mixing them up.

If you aren't comfortable with salads, then switch to smoothies. Start off your day with a few cups of greens, like spinach, with a few chia seeds, banana, nut butter, and almond milk in a blender. You can even add your favorite green supplement to the smoothie, making it a powerful and nutritious drink that your body and hair will love.

Greens like chard, kale, spinach, and collards are by far some of the best vegetables you can have daily to help with hair growth. So drink, juice, and eat up.

TAKEAWAY:

FOR HEALTHY KOILS EAT KALE.

FILTHY WATER CANNOT BE WASHED.

———

West African Proverb

Water Isn't Really Water

LESSON 09

Water is vital to our entire world, but especially our bodies. Water helps to distribute nutrients and vitamins to cells, helps remove toxins from the body, and directly aids hair growth. Unfortunately, most people do not consume the proper amount of water each day, or they have a very hard time drinking enough water. A lot of this has to do with the internal issues going on in the body as well as not having actual pure, clean water. A lot of water that is now offered is enhanced with flavors instead of being filled with loads of oxygen that our body craves.

Did you know that your body strives to maintain a neutral balance of alkalinity and acidity? Foods, water, alcohol, and even stress can and do directly affect a person's overall well-being and also their pH levels. Many studies suggest an acidic body is a magnet for diseases, early aging, and even cancer. Eating more alkaline foods helps shift your body's internal pH and oxygenates your system.

This means your body has more oxygen, which is something our bodies cannot do without every second of the day. Acidic items, such as stomach acid, are needed in order to break down foods, but too many acidic foods internally can hinder and alter our body's pH levels, causing a multitude of health problems. Alkaline foods keep your body healthy and functioning properly and prevent diseases.

What does this have to do with water? If the water or the liquids you consume are more acidic, then this can cause many issues internally, such as acid reflux. Bottled water isn't any good, as most of it is filled with "electrolytes" or "additives" to alter the taste and for other unknown reasons. I recommend that you watch the documentary *Tapped*, which highlights the plastic bottle situation in America.

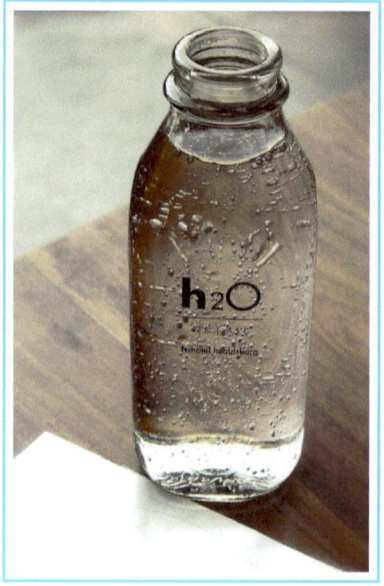

Does this mean we should only drink alkaline water? Eh. I don't drink alkaline water 100 percent of the time because that's unrealistic in my opinion. I am in decent health, and again, I believe in *balance*. If I am running outside and run out of water, I am not going to go around looking for alkaline water. That's unrealistic. I am going to drink fountain water or whatever is available. It's counterproductive for me to pass out from dehydration and then get angry about a huge medical bill that would result from not simply drinking the non-alkaline water. Again, everything in moderation.

This lesson is only here to serve as an eye-opener so you take note of what you eat and drink. Take some time to read labels on bottles and cans. Add a few lemons, limes, or other fruits to your water. Switch it up so that it sparkles. Ditch the soda and artificial juices. Just stay hydrated. But don't over-do it, especially if you are on medication. Again, balance.

TAKEAWAY:

HEALTHY HAIR IS "WATERED" WITH PROPER WATER FROM THE INSIDE AND OUTSIDE.

IF YOU CAN'T EAT OR DRINK IT, THERE IS
A SUPPLEMENT READY FOR YOU TO TAKE.

———

Alexandria Williams

Supplement Heaven or Hell
LESSON 10

Have you looked at the supplement aisle nowadays? Everywhere I go I see supplements literally everywhere. Supplements are a now a billion-dollar industry. From multiple multi-level marketing companies to various vegan supplements, there are a lot of choices. However, when picking a brand, remember the principle in lesson one: *"Whatever the animal ate or the condition of the soil where the fruit/vegetable was planted will be passed along once we consume it."* Once we intake food or water, our body's primary focus is to either store, discard, or process it. So what does this mean for your hair? *It's simple: The condition of the food you're eating will affect what's passed along not just to your hair but also to your entire body.*

The same applies to supplements. *"The FDA is not authorized to review dietary supplement products for safety and effectiveness before they are marketed."*[4] The manufacturers and distributors of dietary supplements are responsible for making sure their products are safe BEFORE they go on to the market.

There have been multiple reports stating that some supplements don't contain the actual ingredients advertised.

CONSUMER REPORT CLAIMS:
Consumers might be attracted to dietary supplements because they're "all natural" and don't contain the synthetic chemicals found in prescription drugs. But they might be getting fooled. In the past two years, according to the Food and Drug Administration, manufacturers have voluntarily recalled more than eighty bodybuilding supplements that contained synthetic steroids or steroid-like substances, fifty sexual-enhancement products that contained sildenafil (Viagra) or other erectile-dysfunction drugs, and forty weight-loss supplements containing sibutramine (Meridia) and other drugs.[5]

There are pros and cons of using supplements. As this book is a basic guideline, I will suggest a few tips on purchasing supplements.

- Review the company's policies and practices regarding supplements.

- Use YouTube videos, Google, Twitter, Amazon, and forums to view real testimonies.

- Talk to local health food store vitamin managers on best supplement brands.

- Look for non-GMO and/or USDA organic labels. If they have both, then it's a winner.

- Review the ingredient list, especially if you have allergies to soy, gluten, and nuts, as many companies use these ingredients in their supplements.

There are tons of supplements everywhere we turn that claim to solve a need or provide a certain element. Supplements, at times, can seem like the new pharmaceutical companies. Many supplements are beneficial, but others are misleading. I can't tell you how many times I have seen "contains soy and gluten and other artificial ingredients" on a multivitamin that claims to be "from real natural whole Food." That title is a bit misleading, don't you think? Be picky with your supplements just as you are with hair products and what goes into your body. It's your body, your money, and your choice.

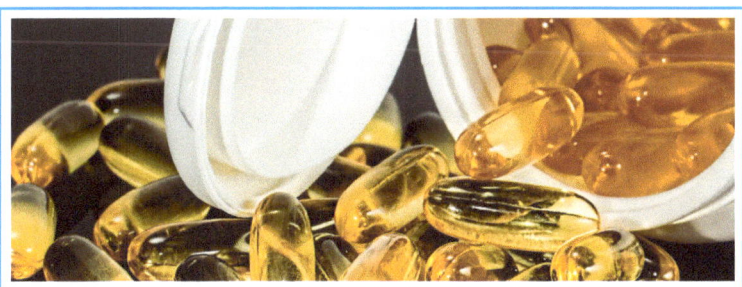

So here is the part I know you've been looking forward to reading. What vitamins or supplements should you take? I love supplements for a variety of reasons, but I still emphasize laying down the proper foundation. Below are a few vitamins that are essential to hair growth.

MULTIVITAMINS:

These contain a variety of necessary vitamins and nutrients needed for daily overall growth. Since many folks don't take in the right amounts of nutrients in a day, multivitamins are a great way to cover the basic vitamins you might be missing. Your multivitamin will contain various vitamins, such as vitamin A, which is an antioxidant that aids in the making of healthy sebum, and Vitamin E, which helps in improving the scalp's circulation. This is a non-negotiable vitamin for me, one each day.

B-COMPLEX:

A B-complex vitamin often contains the B vitamins, which are B1, B2, B3, B5, B6, B7, B9, and B12. These vitamins assist in keeping our bodies running on a daily basis. For example, B12 helps to oxygenate blood vessels, while B6 helps to prevent thinning hair. These vitamins directly affect our energy levels as well as the conversion of food to energy. Not every B-complex vitamin contains similar amounts of equal types of vitamins, nor do they have the same formula. So make sure you compare the amount, sources, and various types of B-complex vitamins.

THE OMEGAS:

I am often amazed at how many people forget the importance of fat and omegas. Fat is vital, as it is brain food. Omega fats play into growing your hair and much more. A proper balance of omegas is essential for our overall health. Lack of the proper amount and ratio of omega fats in your diet could not only cause hair loss issues but also issues in the entire body. For example, a deficiency in omega-3 can cause brittle nails, changes in skin condition, low mental concentration, depression, and much more.

Omega fats help improve your scalp's condition and hair elasticity, and can even assist in the prevention of eczema in some individuals. You can benefit from eating substantial amounts of foods that are rich in omegas, such as salmon, almonds, flax seeds, and avocados. Supplements are also available and have plenty of options, such as fish, hemp, and flaxseed oils supplements.

In the lesson on gut health, I explained the importance of probiotics, so by now you should understand that gut health is the foundation for health and therefore that maintaining good gut health will help your body produce healthy hair.

That is it. These are the basic essentials not just to hair but also to your overall health. Other supplements vary depending on your daily lifestyle needs. "But, Alex, I saw there were some great hair vitamins and this person grew six inches of new hair in just three months of using those vitamins."

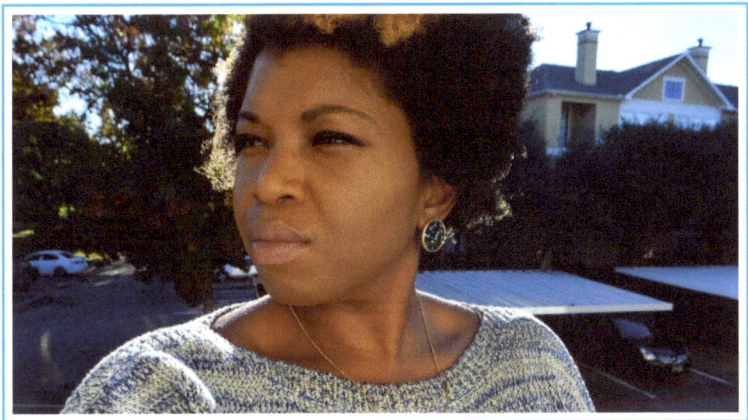

HAIR VITAMINS

Use of hair vitamins has created constant debate in the beauty industry. There are countless hair, skin, and nail vitamins that are being offered in a variety of platforms: Instagram ads, YouTube, and infomercials. Unfortunately, a lot of hair vitamins do more harm than good in my opinion, and their benefits vary based on the individual's health and hair growth cycle. To be blunt, I have checked out several hair vitamins, and most are fancy-marketed B-complex vitamins with added biotin. On top of that, they are filled with a lot of fillers and "artificial ingredients" which can have adverse negative effects.

Not all hair vitamins are bad. Most can enhance your hair growth by helping the body acquire the missing vitamins. Just remember, an overall healthy lifestyle, a balanced diet, and reducing stress is vital for hair growth.

TAKEAWAY:

SUPPLEMENTS FROM REAL FOOD CAN AID IN THE ACHIEVEMENT OF A BALANCED BODY AND FITHAIR.

HEALTHY HAIR IS A BY-PRODUCT OF A
HEALTHY LIFESTYLE.

———

Alexandria Williams

5 Foods for Hair Growth
LESSON 11

Since this book is fairly short, I want to offer some of my top five foods I like that aid in healthy hair growth. Supplements aren't the only way to acquire healthy hair. You can eat your way to a healthy scalp, hair, skin, and body. Here are a few basic foods I have found to aid with hair growth. Eat these daily or weekly to feed your hair from the inside out.

EGGS

Eggs are one of my favorite foods, as they are very cheap and they pack a ton of proteins. One of the benefits of eggs is that they contain biotin and vitamin B12, which are critical for hair growth and aid in better blood circulation. Eggs also contain a variety of minerals, such as iron and zinc, which all play a vital role in overall health and also in growing healthy hair. From boiling to making an egg salad, eggs can easily be integrated into almost any meal.

WILD SALMON

Salmon is a popular fish that is often recommended in dietary plans. It's packed with B vitamins as well as omega-3 fatty acids, which help promote hair growth by keeping your scalp healthy. It also contains vitamin D, which in insufficient amounts can cause hair loss. If possible, try to choose wild salmon, as it contains a bit more nutrients and often has less calories than farm-raised salmon.

SUNFLOWER SEEDS

Sunflower seeds contain vitamin E, which enhances blood flow to the scalp and helps promote faster hair growth. They also contain vitamin B6, which helps address thinning hair. One of the reasons I like sunflower seeds is because they are small, cheap, and can be found almost anywhere. I like to eat them plain or add them to salads.

AVOCADOS

Avocados are a staple in my house. I try to have an avocado daily as one would have an apple. Avocados are filled with essential fatty acids, which are naturally found in skin cells, which help to keep your skin smooth and supple. They can also be applied to the hair and scalp. They have the added ability of stimulating collagen and elastin production.

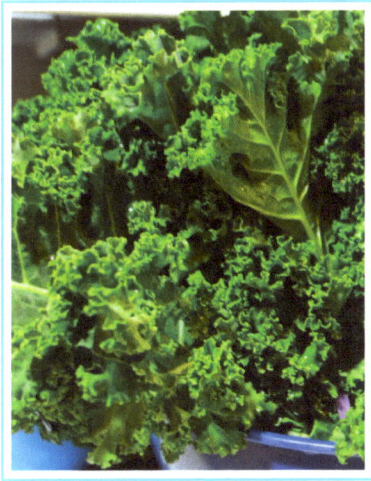

KALE

Kale is one of my favorite green vegetables. If you are following me on social media, then you already know I am obsessed with neon workout gear and kale. From juicing to salads and sandwiches, kale is one of my favorite foods for hair growth, as it contains loads of vitamins and minerals for healthy hair. Kale also has a special place in my heart because I was consistently deficient in iron and decided instead of taking iron pills I would eat a food rich in iron.

The first option was steak, but as a college student, that wasn't an option for me. That is when I learned of a weirdly shaped turnip green vegetable called kale. I learned that this vegetable was higher per calorie in iron than steak/beef and was cheap and low in calories. In addition to kale being an incredibly rich source of iron, it's also high in antioxidants as well as vitamins A and C. These are the things that keep you looking good on the outside but also help grow healthy hair from the inside.

TAKEAWAY:

BE A KALETARIAN.

LET FOOD BE THY MEDICINE AND MEDICINE BE THY FOOD.

———

Hippocrates

Let's Eat

LESSON 12

I am often asked, "What do you eat daily?" Thus I wanted to share a few recipes of my daily favorites. I will make a separate recipe book, but for now, here are a few recipes just to get you started on the FitHair path. There are tons of cookbooks and recipes that inspire me, so make sure you keep up with me on my website, social media, and such. For now, here are a few of my staples:

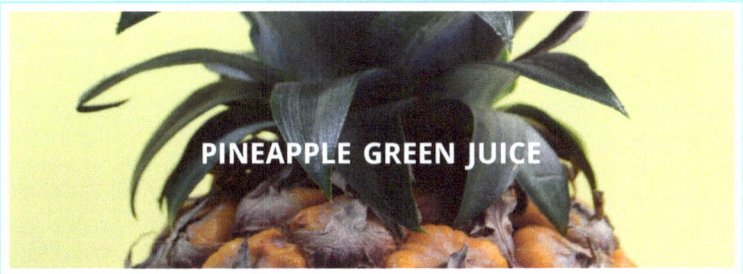

PINEAPPLE GREEN JUICE

- 2 C fresh spinach
- 2 stalks of celery
- 1 pineapple
- 1–2 inches of ginger
- 1–2 limes

Clean ingredients with a fruit and vegetable spray such as Eat Cleaner. Cut and juice all ingredients. Pour and enjoy!

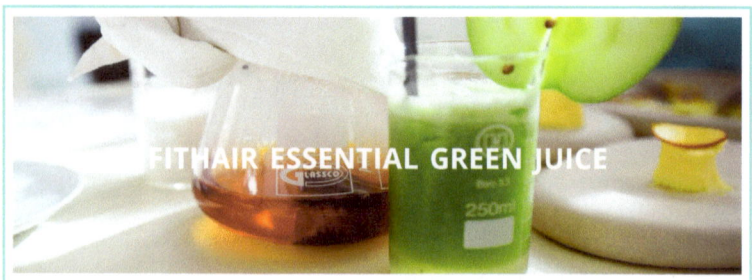

FITHAIR ESSENTIAL GREEN JUICE

- 1-2 green apples
- 2 C of spinach
- 6-8 kale leaves
- 1/2 cucumber
- 2 lemons
- 1-2 inches of ginger

Clean ingredients with a fruit and vegetable spray such as Eat Cleaner. Cut and juice all ingredients. Pour and enjoy!

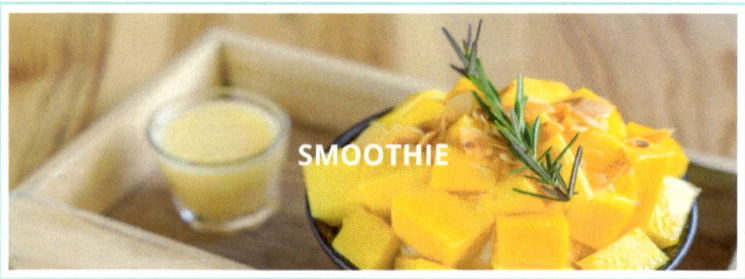

SMOOTHIE

- 1 C of frozen spinach
- 1 handful of fresh kale
- 1 C of mangos
- 2–3 tsp of hemp seeds
- 1 C of almond milk
- 1 scoop of green supplement
- A handful of ice

Blend all ingredients in a blender. Pour and enjoy!

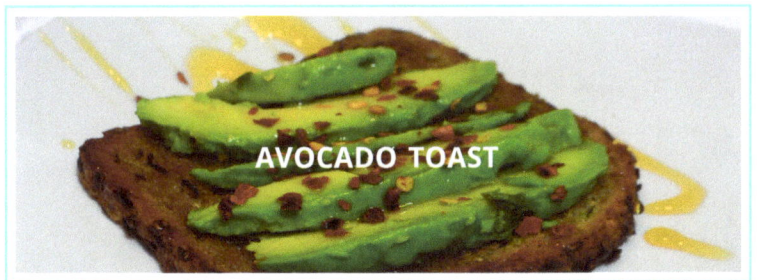

AVOCADO TOAST

- Ezekiel bread
- Avocado
- Half tbsp red pepper flakes
- 1-2 tbsp raw local honey
- Salt and pepper (optional)

Toast bread in toaster or on a grill. Spread avocado on the toast. Drizzle honey on the avocado and toast. Sprinkle some red pepper flakes. Add salt and pepper to taste.

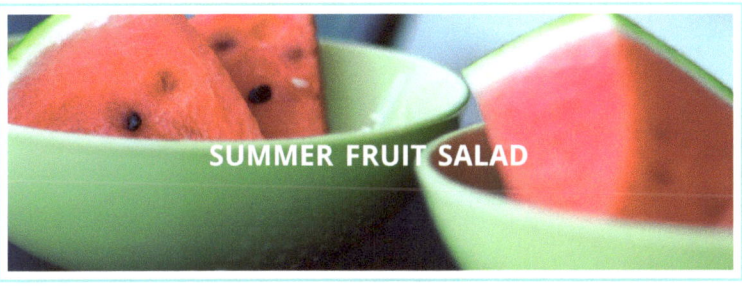

SUMMER FRUIT SALAD

- Pineapple
- Watermelon
- Lime
- 1–2 tbsp of chia seeds

Cut up the pineapple and watermelon into smaller pieces. Add fruit to a bowl. Squeeze juice out of lime. Sprinkle some chia seeds on top. Stir and enjoy.

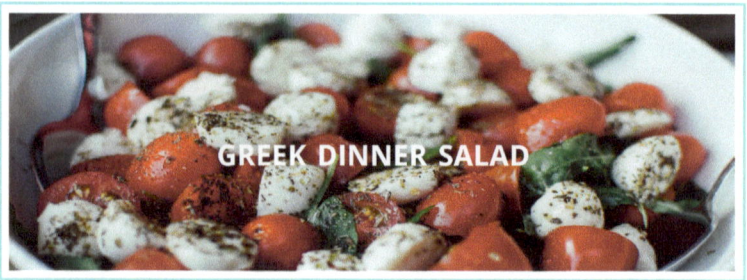

GREEK DINNER SALAD

- Hemp seeds
- Greek yogurt salad dressing
- Grape tomatoes
- Kalamata olives
- Feta cheese

Pour all ingredients into a large salad bowl and mix.

FOOTNOTE

[1] Brain, Marshall. "How Cells Work." How Stuff Works. Accessed December 22, 2016.

[2] Dreher, Christine. "Vitamin Code Story: The Importance of Enzymes." Transform Your Health. Accessed December 22, 2016.

[3] Cross, Joe. "Watch Fat, Sick & Nearly Dead for FREE." Reboot with Joe. January 08, 2016. Accessed December 22, 2016.

[4] FDA "Dietary Supplements: What You Need to Know." FDA Website. January 6, 2016. Accessed December 22, 2016.

[5] "The dangers of dietary and nutritional supplements investigated." Consumer Reports. June 2010. Accessed December 22, 2016.

THERE ARE TONS OF PRODUCTS, FRUITS AND
SUPPLEMENTS ON THE MARKET THAT CAN HELP OR
HINDER YOU HEALTH. BUT THERE ISN'T ANYTHING
IN A BOTTLE OR PILL THAT WILL MAKE YOU
THE PERSON YOU WERE CREATED TO BE.

———

Alexandria Williams

Supplements

LESSON 13

If you have made it this far into to the book, I am giving you a big hug. If you simply flipped to the back of the book, I am still giving you a hug because I made the last chapter dedicated for the folks who just wanted to know what should they go out and by like today.

Here I am summarizing the recommended items I can't live without and recommend. I have used the products for years so I consider them FitHair™ life staples. Don't forget to check my blog, website and social accounts to see the latest stuff recommendations.

SUPPLEMENTS

- Garden of Life My Kind Multi-vitamins
- Country Life Hair Skin & Nails
- Country Life Biotin
- Garden of Life B-Complex
- Nordic Naturals Ultimate Omega D3
- Flora Organic Flax Oil
- Natural Vitality Calm Plus Calcium
- Vega One All-In One
- Burt's Bees Protein + Gut Health
- Burt's Bees Plant-Based Daily Protein
- Nutiva Organic Hemp Protein
- Garden of Life Protein and Greens
- Amazing Grass Green SuperFood
- Vibrant Health Green Vibrance
- Garden of Life Raw Organic Perfect Food
- Garden of Life Dr. Formulated Probiotics

KITCHEN ITEMS

- Santevia
- George Foreman Grill
- Omega Juicers
- Vitamix Blenders
- Blendtec Designer Blenders
- Kleen Kanteen
- NOW Essential Oils

FAVORITE PLACES TO SHOP

- Sprouts Farmers Market
- WholeFoods
- Kroger's

FAVORITE BEAUTY AND HAIR LINES

There are thousands of products on the market and many more to come. I am always trying new items but for now, these product lines are staples. There isn't a product from the following companies that doesn't work for either myself and/or another person.

- Camille Rose Naturals
- Aubrey Organics
- Giovanni Cosmetics
- Dr. Bronner's
- Nubian Heritage
- Avalon Naturals
- Oyin Handmade

If you want to know what's in my bathroom and on my hair. It's going to be on this list.

- Camille Rose Naturals Sweet Ginger Cleaning Rinse
- Camille Rose Naturals Algae Renew Deep Conditioner
- Camille Rose Naturals Almond Jai Twisting Butter
- Camille Rose Naturals Curlaide Moisture Butter
- CURLS Blueberry Bliss Control Jelly
- CURLS Blueberry Bliss Control Paste
- Giovanni 2Chic Ginger and Pineapples Shampoo, Conditioner and Leave-In
- Giovanni Avocado and Olive Oil Deep Conditioner & Hair Mask
- Jane Carter Revitalizing Leave-In Conditioner
- Jane Carter Nourish and Shine
- The Mane Choice- 3-N-1
- The Mane Choice Tropical Moringa Daily Restorative Spray
- The Mane Choice- Crystal Orchid Biotin Infused Styling Gel
- Obia Naturals Curl Hydration Spray
- Silk Elements PURE Oils
- Oyin Handmade Hair Dew
- NOW Sweet Almond Oil
- TGIN Daily Moisturizing cream
- Uncle Funky's Daughters Defunk
- Uncle Funky's Curly Magic Curl Stimulator

Disclaimer

Legal disclaimer

Although the author and publisher have made every effort to ensure that the information in this book was correct at press time, the author and publisher do not assume and hereby disclaim any liability to any party for any loss, damage, or disruption caused by errors or omissions, whether such errors or omissions result from negligence, accident, or any other cause.

This book is not intended as a substitute for the medical advice of physicians. The reader should regularly consult a physician in matters relating to his/her health and particularly with respect to any symptoms that may require diagnosis or medical attention.

Thank you.

Copyright

www.ingramcontent.com/pod-product-compliance
Lightning Source LLC
Chambersburg PA
CBHW040312010626
45792CB00022B/188